FATTY LIVER DIET

50+ Side Dishes, Salad and Pasta recipes designed for Fatty Liver Diet

TABLE OF CONTENTS

Introduction

Fatty liver recipes for personal enjoyment but also for family enjoyment. You will love them for sure for how easy it is to prepare them.

CHICKEN LIVER SALAD

Serves: **4**

Prep Time: **5**   Minutes

Cook Time: **5**   Minutes

Total Time: **10**   Minutes

INGREDIENTS

- 6 thin slices whole meal bread
- 1 orange
- 1 tablespoon olive oil
- 1 lb. chicken liver
- ¼ cup parsley
- ¼ lb. mixed salad leaves

DIRECTIONS

1. In a bowl mix all ingredients and mix well
2. Serve with dressing

Serves: **4**

Prep Time: **5**   Minutes

Cook Time: **5**   Minutes

Total Time: **10**   Minutes

INGREDIENTS

- ¾ head iceberg lettuce
- 1 oz. coriander
- 1 pinch salt
- 2 cloves garlic
- 1 onion
- ¼ tsp curry powder
- 1 lb. chicken livers
- 1 tablespoon olive oil

DIRECTIONS

1. **In a bowl add all ingredients and mix well**
2. **Serve with dressing**

Serves: **2**

Prep Time: **5**   Minutes

Cook Time: **5**   Minutes

Total Time: **10**   Minutes

INGREDIENTS

- 1 onion
- 1 tsp olive oil
- ¼ lb. smoked bacon
- 3 oz. sourdough bread
- 1/3 lb. chicken livers
- 50 ml white wine
- 2 handfuls rocket
- ¼ bunch parsley

DIRECTIONS

1. **In a bowl add all ingredients and mix well**
2. **Serve with dressing**

Serves: **2**

Prep Time: **5**   Minutes

Cook Time: **5**   Minutes

Total Time: **10**   Minutes

INGREDIENTS

- 1 oz. chicken livers
- 1 tsp salt
- 1 slice bread
- 2 tablespoons butter
- 5 rashers bacon
- 3 handfuls of salad leaves

DRESSING

- 1 tablespoon cider vinegar
- 1 tsp mustard
- 1 pinch of salt
- 1 tablespoon live oil
- 1 tablespoon walnut oil

DIRECTIONS

1. In a bowl add all ingredients and mix well
2. Serve with dressing

Serves: *4*
Prep Time: *5*   Minutes

Cook Time: *5*   Minutes

Total Time: *10* Minutes

INGREDIENTS

- 2 red beets
- 1 tablespoon lemon juice
- 1 cup cauliflower florets
- ½ cup vegetable stock
- ½ cup orange juice
- 1 tablespoon unsalted butter
- ¼ cup couscous
- 1 tsp orange zest
- 1 tsp salt

DIRECTIONS

1. In a bowl add all ingredients and mix well
2. Serve with dressing

Serves: **4**

Prep Time: **5**   Minutes

Cook Time: **5**   Minutes

Total Time: **10**   Minutes

INGREDIENTS

- 2 cups vegetable broth
- 2 bay leaves
- ½ cup apple juice
- 1 cup pecans
- 50 ml maple syrup
- 10 Brussels sprouts
- 2 green onions
- 1 pinch salt

DRESSING

- 4 tablespoons olive oil
- 2 tablespoons apple cider vinegar
- 2 tablespoons yeast
- 2 tablespoons maple syrup

DIRECTIONS

1. In a bowl add all ingredients and mix well
2. Serve with dressing

Serves: **2**

Prep Time: **5**   Minutes

Cook Time: **5**   Minutes

Total Time: **10**   Minutes

INGREDIENTS

- 2 boneless chicken breast
- 2 tsp olive oil
- ½ tsp salt
- ½ tsp paprika
- ½ tsp pepper
- ¼ tsp dried basil
- ¼ tsp dried oregano
- 3 cups romaine torn
- 1 tomato
- ½ cup salad dressing

DIRECTIONS

1. In a bowl add all ingredients and mix well
2. Serve with dressing

Serves: **4**

Prep Time: **5**   Minutes

Cook Time: **5**   Minutes

Total Time: **10** Minutes

INGREDIENTS

- 1 orange
- 1 lemon
- 1 lime
- 1 pink grapefruit
- 1/3 baby arugula
- ½ lb. feta
- 2 onions
- 1 tablespoon sesame seeds

DRESSING

- juice of 1 lime
- juice of 1 orange
- 1 tablespoon honey
- 1 tablespoon white vinegar
- 1/3 cup olive oil

DIRECTIONS

1. In a bowl add all ingredients and mix well
2. Serve with dressing

Serves: **4**

Prep Time: **5**   Minutes

Cook Time: **5**   Minutes

Total Time: **10**   Minutes

INGREDIENTS

- 1 oakleaf lettuce
- 3 ripe figs
- ¼ lb. prosciutto
- 12 basil leaves
- 2 oz. parmesan

ORANGE VINAIGRETTE

- 1 tablespoon orange juice
- 1 tsp balsamic vinegar
- 1 tsp mustard
- ¼ tsp orange zest
- ½ cup olive oil

DIRECTIONS

1. In a bowl add all ingredients and mix well
2. Serve with dressing

Serves: *4*

Prep Time: 5   Minutes

Cook Time: 5   Minutes

Total Time: *10*   Minutes

INGREDIENTS

- 1 carrot
- ½ red cabbage
- 1 handful parsley
- 2 scallions
- 2 tablespoon mayonnaise
- salt

DIRECTIONS

1. In a bowl add all ingredients and mix well
2. Serve with dressing

Serves: **4**

Prep Time: **5**   Minutes

Cook Time: **5**   Minutes

Total Time: ***10***   Minutes

INGREDIENTS

- ½ cup pine nuts
- ¼ apple
- ¾ cup blue cheese
- 6 oz. salad greens

DRESSING

- 1 tsp Dijon mustard
- 2 tablespoons balsamic vinegar
- ¼ cup olive oil
- 1 heaping tablespoon fig jam
- 1 garlic clove

DIRECTIONS

1. In a bowl add all ingredients and mix well
2. Serve with dressing

Serves: **4**

Prep Time: **5**   Minutes

Cook Time: **5**   Minutes

Total Time: **10**   Minutes

INGREDIENTS

- 2 cans white beans
- 2 cloves garlic
- 1 onion
- ¼ cup parsley
- 2 tablespoons olive oil
- 2 tomatoes
- ½ cup black olives
- 2 tablespoons wine vinegar
- lemon juice for 1 lemon
- 1 pinch of salt

DIRECTIONS

1. In a bowl add all ingredients and mix well
2. Serve with dressing

Serves: **4**

Prep Time: **5**   Minutes

Cook Time: **5**   Minutes

Total Time: **10**   Minutes

INGREDIENTS

- ½ cup miso
- 1 tablespoon rice vinegar
- 1 tablespoon soy sauce
- 1 tablespoon sesame oil
- ¼ tsp ginger
- 1 tablespoon water

DIRECTIONS

1. In a bowl add all ingredients and mix well
2. Serve with dressing

Serves: **4**

Prep Time: **5**   Minutes

Cook Time: **5**   Minutes

Total Time: **10**   Minutes

INGREDIENTS

- 1 head roasted cauliflower
- 1 tablespoon canola
- 1 tsp turmeric
- 1 tsp cumin
- 1 pinch of salt
- ½ red onion
- 1 tablespoon lemon juice
- 1 tsp honey
- ½ cup pomegranate seeds
- 2 heaping tablespoons parsley

DIRECTIONS

1. In a bowl add all ingredients and mix well
2. Serve with dressing

Serves: **4**

Prep Time: **5**   Minutes

Cook Time: **5**   Minutes

Total Time: **10**   Minutes

INGREDIENTS

- 10 bacon
- 2 broccoli crowns
- 1 red onion
- ¼ cup raisins

DRESSING

- 1 cup mayonnaise
- 1 tablespoon balsamic vinegar
- 1 tsp sugar

DIRECTIONS

1. In a bowl add all ingredients and mix well
2. Serve with dressing

Serves: **4**

Prep Time: **5**   Minutes

Cook Time: **5**   Minutes

Total Time: **10**   Minutes

INGREDIENTS

- 1 lb. red potatoes
- 3 eggs
- 2 ribs celery
- ¼ cup red onion
- 3 green onions
- 2 tablespoons diced dill pickle
- ½ cup sour cream
- 1/3 cup mayonnaise
- 1 tablespoon tarragon vinegar
- 1 tsp mustard
- ¼ tsp salt
- ¼ tsp pepper

DIRECTIONS

1. In a bowl add all ingredients and mix well
2. Serve with dressing

Serves: *4*

Prep Time: *5*   Minutes

Cook Time: *5*   Minutes

Total Time: *10*   Minutes

INGREDIENTS

- 1 cup mayonnaise
- 2 tablespoons sugar
- 2 tablespoons apple cider vinegar
- 1 head red cabbage
- 1 red onion
- 1/3 cup raisins
- 3 tablespoons pecans

DIRECTIONS

1. In a bowl add all ingredients and mix well
2. Serve with dressing

PIZZA RECIPES

GRAIN-FREE PIZZA CRUST

Serves: *4*

Prep Time: *15*   Minutes

Cook Time: *15*   Minutes

Total Time: *30*   Minutes

INGREDIENTS

- 2 eggs
- 2 tablespoons apple sauce
- ¼ cup coconut flour
- ½ cup almond flour
- ½ tsp salt
- ½ tsp dried basil

DIRECTIONS

1. In a food processor add the eggs and process until smooth
2. Add salt, coconut flour, applesauce, almond flour and mix well
3. Mix until it forms a ball in the processor

4. Scrap the dough together into a ball, put the dough onto the parchment paper

5. Bake at 350 F for 15 minutes

6. Remove from oven and serve the pizza crust

Serves: **4**

Prep Time: **10**   Minutes

Cook Time: **20**   Minutes

Total Time: **30**   Minutes

INGREDIENTS

- ½ cup water
- 1 envelope active dry yeast
- 1 cup water
- 1 tablespoon olive oil
- 3 cups bread flour
- 1 tsp salt
- 1 tsp vegetable oil

DIRECTIONS

1. Sprinkle water in yeast and let it stand for a couple of minutes
2. Add oil and stir to combine
3. In a blender add flour and salt and blend for 30-45 seconds
4. Pour liquid ingredients and continue to blend until it the dough is formed

5. Put dough into an oiled bowl, cover and let it stand for 1-2 hours

6. Over dough add toppings like, red pepper flakes, onion, olives, chicken livers and cheddar cheese

7. Preheat the oven at 475 F

8. Bake pizza for 15-18 minutes or until golden brown

9. When ready remove and serve

Serves: *4*

Prep Time: *10*   Minutes

Cook Time: *20*   Minutes

Total Time: *30*   Minutes

INGREDIENTS

- ½ head cauliflower
- 1 tablespoon almond meal
- 1 tsp oregano
- 1 egg

SAUCE

- 1 tomato
- 1 head garlic
- 1 handful basil
- 1 drizzle olive oil

DIRECTIONS

1. Preheat the oven at 325 F

2. In a blender add chopped cauliflower and blend for 60 seconds, place it in a bowl and microwave for 4-5 minutes

3. Add the rest of the ingredients to the bowl and mix well

4. Spread mixture on a cookie sheet lined with parchment paper and bake for 12-15 minutes

5. In a blender add all ingredients for the sauce and blend until smooth

6. Add to your pan on the stove and cook

7. Add toppings like red pepper, mushrooms, zucchini, spinach

8. Bake for another 8-10 minutes

9. When ready remove and serve

Serves: **4**

Prep Time: **10**   Minutes

Cook Time: **20**   Minutes

Total Time: **30**   Minutes

INGREDIENTS

- 1 lb. ground beef
- 1 egg
- 1 tsp parsley
- 1 tsp dried basil
- ¼ tsp salt
- ½ tsp pepper
- ¼ cup tomato puree
- 1 tsp tomato paste
- ¼ red pepper
- 1 tsp dried basil
- ¼ cup olives
- 5 slices prosciutto
- 4 oz. parmesan
- 1 handful fresh basil

DIRECTIONS

1. Preheat the oven to 430 F
2. In a bowl add salt, mince, egg, basil, pepper, parsley and mix well
3. Roll into a ball and place on a baking tray
4. Bake for 12-15 minutes
5. Mix the tomato paste with tomato puree and spread across the base
6. Top with peppers, prosciutto, parmesan, olives and bake for another 8-10 minutes
7. Remove from the oven, top with basil leaves and serve

Serves: **4**

Prep Time: **10** Minutes

Cook Time: **20** Minutes

Total Time: **30** Minutes

INGREDIENTS

- 1 gluten-free pizza crust

SAUCE

- 1 tablespoons tomato paste
- 1 tablespoon balsamic vinegar
- 1 tsp honey
- 1 clove garlic

TOPPINGS

- 1 tsp olive oil
- ¼ onion
- 1 cup shiitake mushrooms
- ¼ bell pepper
- ½ cup jarred artichokes
- 1 tablespoon sun-dried tomatoes

-   1 tablespoon balsamic vinegar

DIRECTIONS

1. Preheat the oven to 350 F
2. Cook your pizza crust fro 12-15 minutes
3. In a pan add olive oil, mushrooms and the rest of the toppings and cook for 5-7 minutes on low heat
4. In a bowl prepare add all the ingredients for the sauce and mix well
5. Remove pizza crust from the oven, add pizza sauce and toppings
6. Place pizza back in the oven and bake for 8-10 minutes
7. When ready, remove and serve

Serves: **4**

Prep Time: **10**   Minutes

Cook Time: **30**   Minutes

Total Time: **40**   Minutes

INGREDIENTS

- 1 cauliflower head
- 1 cup parmesan
- ¼ tsp Italian seasoning
- 1 clove garlic
- ¼ tsp salt
- 1 egg
- olive oil
- 1 cup mozzarella
- ¼ cup marinara sauce
- ½ cup basil leaves
- 1 tomato

DIRECTIONS

1. **Preheat the oven to 450 F**

2. In a blender add cauliflower and blend until finely ground

3. In a bowl add parmesan, cauliflower, garlic, egg, Italian seasoning, salt and mix well

4. Spread the cauliflower mixture on a parchment paper and bake until the crust is barely golden, 12-15 minutes

5. Remove from the oven, sprinkle with mozzarella, marinara sauce, tomato slices and bake for another 6-8 minutes

6. When ready, remove and serve

Serves: **2**

Prep Time: **10** Minutes

Cook Time: **30** Minutes

Total Time: **40** Minutes

INGREDIENTS

- 1 cup gluten-free flour
- 1 tsp psllium husk powder
- ½ tsp salt
- ¼ tsp active dry yeast
- ¼ tsp olive oil
- ¾ cup water
- 2 cups lentil hummus
- 7 slices eggplant
- 4 sweet peppers sliced
- 6 olives sliced

DIRECTIONS

1. Preheat the oven at 350 F
2. In a bowl whisk psyllium husk, yeast, salt, flour and mix well

3. Add olive oil, water, mix and let the dough rise for 2-3 hours

4. Transfer the dough onto a surface and roll the dough to form a smooth ball and then flatten the ball to form a disk

5. Fold the pizza dough disk in half, and then again, form a triangle

6. Transfer onto a dusted pizza pan

7. Bake for 15-18 minutes or until barely golden

8. Remove from the oven, spoon the lentil hummus in the center, eggplant slices, olives, peppers and sprinkle with cheese on top

9. Bake for another 6-8 minutes

10. When ready remove and serve

Serves: **4**

Prep Time: **10**   Minutes

Cook Time: **35**   Minutes

Total Time: **45**   Minutes

INGREDIENTS

CRUST

- 1/2 butternut squash
- 1 garlic clove
- 1 tablespoon ground flaxseed
- ¾ cup flaxseed
- 1 tsp salt
- 1 tsp thyme

SQUASH HUMMUS

- 2 cups butternut squash
- 1 cup raw walnuts
- 1 tsp thyme
- 1 garlic clove
- 2 tsp cumin
- water as needed
- spinach leaves

- 6 tomato slices

DIRECTIONS

1. Preheat the oven to 375 F
2. In a blender add all ingredients for the crust and blend until smooth
3. Add water if necessary and blend again
4. Spread batter into a circle on a lined dehydrator tray and dehydrate for 16-18 hours
5. For squash mush combine all ingredients and blend until smooth
6. Spread the hummus over the crust and top with tomatoes, onion, spinach leaves
7. When ready, serve!

Serves: **4**

Prep Time: **10**   Minutes

Cook Time: **30**   Minutes

Total Time: **40**   Minutes

INGREDIENTS

- 4 zucchini
- 2 tsp salt
- 2 cups almond flour
- 2 tablespoons coconut flour
- 3 eggs
- 2 ½ cups parmesan cheese
- 1 tsp red pepper flakes
- 1 tsp dried oregano

DIRECTIONS

1. Shred the zucchini, sprinkle with salt and set aside
2. Preheat the oven to 400 F
3. Mix zucchini with remaining ingredients
4. Place the dough over a baking sheet and spread evenly

5. Pop the pizza crust in the oven for 30 minutes or until golden brown

6. When ready, remove and serve

Serves: *4*

Prep Time: *10*   Minutes

Cook Time: *20*   Minutes

Total Time: *30*   Minutes

INGREDIENTS

CRUST
- ½ cup hemp seeds
- 1 cup walnuts
- 1 tsp salt
- 1 tsp basil
- 1 tablespoon maple syrup
- 1 tablespoon water
- ¼ onion

PESTO
- 4 cups spinach
- ¼ cup pine nuts
- 1 garlic clove
- ¼ tsp salt
- ¼ cup water

TOPPINGS
- 3-4 mushrooms

- 1 bell pepper
- 1 tomato
- 1 tsp tamari

DIRECTIONS

1. In a blender add all ingredients for the crust and blend until smooth
2. Spread batter into a circle on a lined dehydrator tray and dehydrate for 4-5 hours
3. In a blender add all ingredients for pesto and blend until it reaches pesto consistency
4. Spread pesto over pizza crust and add toppings
5. When ready, serve

Serves: *4*

Prep Time: *10*   Minutes

Cook Time: *30*   Minutes

Total Time: *40*   Minutes

INGREDIENTS

- cashew cheese as needed
- tomato sauce as needed

CRUST

- 6 tomatoes
- 1 zucchini pulp
- 1 red bell pepper
- 1 onion
- 1 tablespoon flax seeds
- 2 tablespoon sesame seeds
- 1 tablespoon ground sunflower seeds
- 1 tablespoon tamari sauce
- 1 tablespoon olive oil

TOPPINGS

- arugula
- 4-5 cherry tomatoes

- 3-4 mushrooms
- 4-5 black olives

DIRECTIONS

1. In a blender add all ingredients for the crust and blend until smooth
2. Spread batter into a circle on a lined dehydrator tray and dehydrate for 10-12 hours
3. Cut the ingredients for toppings in thin slices
4. Place tomato sauce, cashew cheese and toppings over pizza crust
5. Serve when ready

SIDE DISHES

SESAME PORK TACOS

Serves: **4**

Prep Time: **5**   Minutes

Cook Time: **15**   Minutes

Total Time: **25**   Minutes

INGREDIENTS

- 1 cup cucumber slices
- 5 radishes
- ½ cup red wine vinegar
- 3 tsp sugar
- 1 tablespoon olive oil
- 3 scallions
- 1 cup red cabbage
- 1 lb. ground pork
- 2 tsp garlic powder
- 2 tablespoons sesame oil
- 2 tablespoons soy sauce
- 1 tsp Sriracha
- 10 tortillas
- 1 tsp cilantro

- ¼ cup sour cream
- 1 pinch of salt

DIRECTIONS

1. In a bowl add radishes, cucumbers, vinegar, 1 tsp sugar and salt, stir well to combine
2. In a pan add oil, scallions, cabbage and cook for 4-5 minutes
3. Add pork, sugar, garlic powder and cook for another 4-5 minutes
4. Add soy sauce, sesame oil and stir to combine
5. Spread sour cream in the center of your tortilla, add pork filling and sprinkle cilantro, radishes and top with meat mixture

Serves: *3*
Prep Time: *10*   Minutes

Cook Time: *10*   Minutes

Total Time: *20*   Minutes

INGREDIENTS

- 2 cups ripe watermelon
- 1 red pepper
- ¼ onion
- 3 tablespoons red wine vinegar
- 6 tablespoons cranberry juice
- Italian basil leaves as needed

DIRECTIONS

1. Puree all ingredients, except the basil, until smooth
2. Refrigerate to chill
3. Serve garnished with basil, onion, tomato or cucumber

Serves: **5**

Prep Time: **10**   Minutes

Cook Time: **40**   Minutes

Total Time: **50**   Minutes

INGREDIENTS

- 1 tablespoon olive oil
- ¾ cup onion
- 2 ½ cups water
- 2 cups zucchini
- 1 cup sliced carrots
- 1 cup beans
- ¼ cup celery
- 2 tablespoons basil
- 1/3 tsp oregano
- ¼ tsp salt
- ¼ tsp black pepper
- 1 can plum tomatoes
- 2 cloves garlic
- ½ cup uncooked pasta

DIRECTIONS

1. In a saucepan add oil, onion and sauté for 4-5 minutes

2. Add remaining ingredients and bring to a boil

3. Reduce heat and simmer on low heat for 20-25 minutes

4. Add pasta and cook until pasta is al dente for 10-12 minutes

5. When ready, remove from heat and serve

Serves: **3**

Prep Time: **5**   Minutes

Cook Time: **15** Minutes

Total Time: **20** Minutes

INGREDIENTS

- 3 ears of corn
- 2 tablespoons mayonnaise
- 2 tablespoons squeezed lime juice
- ½ tsp chili powder
- 1 pinch of salt

DIRECTIONS

1. Place corn onto the grill and cook for 5-6 minutes or until the kernels being to brown
2. Turn every few minutes until all sides are slightly charred
3. In a bowl mix the rest of ingredients
4. Spread a light coating of the mixture onto each cob and serve

Serves: **4**

Prep Time: **10** Minutes

Cook Time: **30** Minutes

Total Time: **40** Minutes

INGREDIENTS

- 6 oz. squash
- ½ bunch basil
- ¼ cup macadamia nuts
- 1 tablespoon olive oil
- ¼ lemon
- ¼ tsp ground smoked paprika
- salt
- vegetable sticks

DIRECTIONS

1. Preheat the oven to 350 F
2. Cut the squash into chunks and roast for 25-30 minutes
3. In a food processor add the basil leaves, lemon zest, macadamia nuts, squash pieces and salt

4. Serve with vegetable sticks: cucumber, carrots, tomatoes and green pepper

Serves: **6**

Prep Time: **10**   Minutes

Cook Time: **15**   Minutes

Total Time: **25**   Minutes

INGREDIENTS

- 1 cup white whole wheat flour
- 1 cornstarch
- 1 tsp baking powder
- 1 tsp ground ginger
- ½ tsp ground cinnamon
- ¼ tsp nutmeg
- ¼ tsp ground cloves
- ½ tsp salt
- 1 tablespoon unsalted butter
- 1 egg white
- 2 tsp vanilla stevia
- ½ cup nonfat milk
- ½ cup molasses
- 1 tsp vanilla extract

DIRECTIONS

1. Preheat the oven to 350 F

2. In a bowl whisk together the cornstarch, ginger, baking powder, cinnamon, nutmeg, cloves and salt and flour

3. In another bowl mix vanilla extract, egg, butter, stevia, molasses and milk

4. Add in the flour mixture and stir until fully incorporated

5. Divide dough into 14-16 portions and roll each into a ball

6. Place onto a baking sheet and press it down into the cookie dough

7. Bake for 8-10 minutes

8. When ready, remove and serve

Serves: **4**

Prep Time: **10**   Minutes

Cook Time: **40**   Minutes

Total Time: **50**   Minutes

INGREDIENTS

- 4 red bell peppers
- 1 lb. ground turkey
- 1 tablespoon olive oil
- ¼ onion
- 1 cup mushrooms 1 zucchini
- ½ green bell pepper
- ½ yellow bell pepper
- 1 cup spinach
- 1 can diced tomatoes
- 1 tsp Italian seasoning
- ¼ tsp garlic powder
- 1 pinch of salt

DIRECTIONS

1. **Preheat the oven to 325 F**

2. In a pot bring water to boil, add pepper and cook for 5-6 minutes

3. In a skillet cook the turkey until brown and set aside

4. In another pan add onion, olive oil, mushrooms, zucchini, green, yellow pepper, spinach and cook until tender

5. Add remaining ingredients to the turkey and cook until done

6. Stuff the peppers with the mixture and place them into a casserole dish

7. Bake for 15-18 minutes or until done

Serves: **6**

Prep Time: **10**   Minutes

Cook Time: **50**   Minutes

Total Time: **60**   Minutes

INGREDIENTS

- 1 cup red quinoa
- 1 cup vegetable broth
- ¾ cup water

SEASONING

- ¼ cup salsa
- 1 tablespoon yeast
- 1 tsp cumin
- 1 tsp chili powder
- ¼ tsp garlic powder
- ½ tsp black pepper
- ½ tsp salt
- 1 tablespoon olive oil
-

DIRECTIONS

1. **In a saucepan add quinoa and cook for 5-6 minutes**

2. Add water, vegetable broth and bring to a boil
3. Reduce heat to low and cook for 20-22 minutes or until liquid is absorbed
4. Add quinoa to a mixing bowl, remaining ingredients and toss to combine
5. Bake for 25-30 minutes or until golden brown
6. When ready remove and serve with taco salads, enchiladas or nachos

Serves: **6**

Prep Time: **10** Minutes

Cook Time: **25** Minutes

Total Time: **35** Minutes

INGREDIENTS

- 1 bunch of kale
- 1 tablespoon olive oil
- 1 tsp salt

DIRECTIONS

1. Preheat the oven to 325 F
2. Chop the kale into chip size pieces
3. Put pieces into a bowl tops with olive oil and salt
4. Spread the leaves in a single layer onto a parchment paper
5. Bake for 20-25 minutes
6. When ready, remove and serve

Serves: **2**

Prep Time: **10**   Minutes

Cook Time: **15**   Minutes

Total Time: **25**   Minutes

INGREDIENTS

- 1 cup cooked rice pasta
- 1 chicken breast
- ¼ cup no sugar marinara sauce
- ½ cup tomatoes
- parsley for serving
- 1 tsp olive oil

DIRECTIONS

1. In a skillet cook the pasta according to the package directions
2. Drain and rinse the pasta
3. Add cooked chicken breast, marinara sauce and serve

Serves: **4**
Prep Time: **5**   Minutes
Cook Time: **20**   Minutes
Total Time: **25**   Minutes

INGREDIENTS

- 2 tsp olive oil
- 1 onion
- 3 portobello mushrooms
- 1 red bell pepper
- 1 tsp dried oregano
- ¼ tsp ground pepper
- 1 tablespoon all-purpose flour
- ½ cup vegetable broth
- 1 tablespoon soy sauce
- 2 oz. vegan cheese
- 3 whole-wheat rolls

DIRECTIONS

1. In a skillet add onion, pepper, bell pepper, oregano and cook until soft

2. Reduce heat, sprinkle flour, soy sauce, broth and bring to a simmer

3. Remove from heat, add cheese slices on top and let it stand until fully melted

4. Divide into 3-4 portions and serve

Serves: **4**
Prep Time: **10** Minutes

Cook Time: **50** Minutes

Total Time: **60** Minutes

INGREDIENTS

- 1 head cauliflower
- ¼ unsweetened almond milk
- ¼ cup water
- ¾ rice flour
- 1 tsp garlic powder
- 1 tsp onion powder
- 1 tsp cumin
- 1 tsp paprika
- ½ tsp salt
- ¼ tsp ground pepper
- bbq sauce

VINEGAR SAUCE

- 1 tablespoon vegan butter
- 2 tablespoons apple cider vinegar

- 1 tablespoon water
- 1 pinch of salt

DIRECTIONS

1. Preheat the oven to 425 F
2. Mix all wing ingredients in a bowl and submerge each cauliflower floret into the mix
3. Place florets on a prepare baking sheet
4. Bake for 10 minutes, flip and bake for another 10 minutes or until golden brown
5. Remove the cauliflower from the oven and serve with vinegar sauce
6. When ready season with pepper and salt and serve

Serves: **4**

Prep Time: 5   Minutes

Cook Time: **15**   Minutes

Total Time: **20**   Minutes

INGREDIENTS

- 5 heads baby bok choy
- olive oil
- 1 tsp pepper
- 1 tsp salt

DIRECTIONS

1. Preheat the oven to 425 F
2. Cut each bok choy in half lengthwise and place on a baking sheet
3. Drizzle with olive oil, pepper and salt
4. Bake for 10-12 minutes, flip and bake for another 8-10 minutes
5. When ready remove and serve

Serves: *12*
Prep Time: *10*   Minutes

Cook Time: *120*   Minutes

Total Time: *130*   Minutes

INGREDIENTS

- 12 lbs. turkey
- 4 tablespoons melted
- 1 tsp pepper
- salt as needed

DIRECTIONS

1. Preheat the oven at 400 F
2. Prepare the turkey to be roasted
3. Brush the breast and legs of the turkey with butter, salt, pepper and arrange it breast-side down on a rack
4. Roast for 60-75 minutes
5. Remove from the oven, tip the juice from the cavity of the turkey into the pan
6. Flip the turkey breast-side up and place back in the oven at 375 F for another 60 minutes

7. When ready, remove and serve

Serves: *12*
Prep Time: *10* Minutes

Cook Time: *50* Minutes

Total Time: *60* Minutes

INGREDIENTS

- ½ cup maple syrup
- 1 tablespoon butter
- 1 tablespoon lemon juice
- ¼ tsp salt
- 2 lbs. sweet potatoes
- 1 red onion

DIRECTIONS

1. Preheat the oven to 425 F
2. In a bowl combine butter, lemon juice, maple syrup, salt and pepper
3. Place sweet potatoes and onions into a baking dish
4. Pour maple syrup mixture over the potatoes and bake for 12-15 minutes or until golden brown
5. When ready, remove and and serve

Serves: *8*

Prep Time: *10*   Minutes

Cook Time: *30*   Minutes

Total Time: *40*   Minutes

INGREDIENTS

- 1 head of cauliflower
- ¼ tsp chili powder
- 2 cloves garlic
- 2 tablespoons cilantro
- 1 tsp salt
- ¼ tsp black pepper
- 2 eggs
- 3 tablespoons cornmeal
- ½ cup flour
- 4 tablespoons nutritional yeast

DIRECTIONS

1. Cook cauliflower florets by steaming for 5-6 minutes
2. Mix the cauliflower with chili powder, cilantro, garlic, pepper and salt

3. In another bowl beat the egg, add cauliflower mixture, flour, corn meal and yeast
4. Add ¼ cup of the mixture to the pan and press down the fritter
5. Cook until golden brown for 3-4 minutes per side
6. When ready, remove and serve

PEACH CRUMBLE

Serves: **8**

Prep Time: **10**   Minutes

Cook Time: **40**   Minutes

Total Time: **50**   Minutes

INGREDIENTS

- 3 peaches
- 2 tablespoons cornstarch
- 1 tsp almond extract
- 1 tsp cinnamon
- ¾ cup old-fashioned oats
- ½ cup whole wheat flour
- 2 tablespoons agave

DIRECTIONS

1. Preheat the oven to 325 F
2. In a bowl mix cornstarch, almond extract, peaches and ½ cinnamon
3. In another bowl mix flour, oats and remaining cinnamon
4. Add in agave and mix well

5. Spread mixture into a baking dish and sprinkle oat crumbs on top

6. Bake for 35-40 minutes or until mixture turns crunchy

7. When ready remove and serve

Serves: **6**

Prep Time: **10**   Minutes

Cook Time: **90**   Minutes

Total Time: **100** Minutes

INGREDIENTS

- ½ cup olive oil
- 1 eggplant
- 1 onion
- 2 garlic cloves
- 1 lb. potatoes
- 5 tomatoes
- 10 cherry tomatoes
- 1 cup tomato passata
- 1 cup water
- 1 tablespoon dried oregano
- 1 tablespoon parsley
- 1 tsp salt

DIRECTIONS

1. **Preheat the oven to 400 F**

2. In a frying pan add olive oil, eggplant and cook for 6-7 minutes

3. Add garlic, onion and sauté for 5-6 minutes

4. Add potato, zucchini, passata, tomatoes and water

5. Sprinkle with oregano, parley, pepper and salt

6. Mix well and transfer to a baking dish, drizzle with olive oil and bake for 45-55 minutes or until the top has browned

7. When ready remove and serve

Serves: **4**

Prep Time: **5** Minutes

Cook Time: **15** Minutes

Total Time: **20** Minutes

INGREDIENTS

- 1 lb. chicken meat
- 2 cups bread crumbs
- ½ cup low-fat milk
- 2 tablespoons grated onion
- ¼ tsp black pepper
- ¼ tsp salt
- 1 tsp olive oil

DIRECTIONS

1. Place chicken in a bowl and fold in bread crumbs, cayenne, onion, salt and pepper
2. Divide chicken meat into 4 piles and shape into patties
3. Coat each patty with bread crumbs
4. Fry the patty for 4-5 per side or until golden

5. When ready remove and serve

Serves: **8**

Prep Time: **10** Minutes

Cook Time: **90** Minutes

Total Time: **100** Minutes

INGREDIENTS

- ¼ cup oats
- ½ cup milk
- 1 onion
- 2 lbs. ground turkey breast
- ½ cup red bell pepper
- 2 eggs
- 2 tsp Worcestershire sauce
- ½ cup ketchup
- ¼ tsp salt
- 1 can tomato sauce

DIRECTIONS

1. Preheat the oven to 375 F
2. In a bowl stir in oats milk and let it soak for a couple of minutes

84

3. In another bowl combine the ingredients except tomato sauce
4. Transfer the mixture to a baking dish and shape into a loaf
5. Pour tomato sauce over the meatloaf
6. Bake for 60 minutes
7. When ready remove and serve

PASTA & NOODLES

ROASTED CHICKPEAS

Serves: **6**

Prep Time: **5**   Minutes

Cook Time: **50**   Minutes

Total Time: **55**   Minutes

INGREDIENTS

- 2 cans chickpeas
- ¼ tsp salt
- 2 tablespoons olive oil

DIRECTIONS

1. Preheat the oven to 400 F
2. Place the chickpeas on a baking sheet and toss with olive oil until they are coated
3. Sprinkle with salt and spread the chickpeas out
4. Bake for 45-55 minutes or until crispy
5. When ready remove and serve

Serves: **4**

Prep Time: **10**   Minutes

Cook Time: **15**   Minutes

Total Time: **25**   Minutes

INGREDIENTS

- 1 tsp salt
- 1 lb. ground chicken
- 2 cloves garlic
- ¼ onion
- ½ cup hoisin sauce
- 1 tablespoon soy sauce
- 1 tablespoon wine vinegar
- 1 tablespoon ginger
- 1 tsp Sriracha
- 1 can chestnuts
- 2 green onion
- 1 carrot
- 1 heat butter lettuce

DIRECTIONS

1. In a saucepan add olive oil, ground chicken and cook for 4-5 minutes

2. Stir in onion, garlic, hoisin sauce, wine vinegar, soy sauce, ginger, Sriracha until onions are translucent

3. Stir in water chestnuts and season with salt and pepper

4. When ready spoon chicken mixture into the center of a lettuce leaf and top with carrot

Serves: **6**
Prep Time: **20**   Minutes

Cook Time: **60**   Minutes

Total Time: **80**   Minutes

INGREDIENTS

- 1 tsp coconut oil
- ¼ cup onion
- 1 cup brown rice
- ½ cup golden raisins
- 1 tsp fresh turmeric
- 2 cloves garlic
- 2 cups vegetable broth
- 1 pinch of salt

DIRECTIONS

1. In a saucepan add coconut oil, onions and sauce for 4-5 minutes
2. Add raisins, turmeric, rice and garlic, toss to coat
3. Sauté for 2-3 minutes and slowly bring saucepan to a boil

4. Reduce heat and cook for 40-45 minutes or until rice is tender

5. When ready season with salt, pepper and serve

Serves: *3*
Prep Time: *10*   Minutes

Cook Time: *15*   Minutes

Total Time: *25*   Minutes

INGREDIENTS

- 2 beets
- olive oil
- 2 cups baby kale

PESTO

- 2 cups basil leaves
- ½ cup Pinenuts
- ½ cup olive oil
- ¼ tsp salt
- ½ tsp pepper
- 1 clove garlic

DIRECTIONS

1. **Preheat the oven to 400 F**

2. On a baking sheet spread out the beet noodles and bake for 8-10 minutes

3. In a bowl mix all pesto ingredients and place in a blender, blend until smooth

4. Toss beets with pesto, kale and serve

Serves: **5**

Prep Time: **10**   Minutes

Cook Time: **30**   Minutes

Total Time: **40**   Minutes

INGREDIENTS

- 2 zucchini
- 1 avocado
- 1 handful basil
- juice from ½ lemon
- 1 garlic clove
- 2 tablespoons olive oil
- 1 tablespoon water
- 1 tsp salt

DIRECTIONS

1. Make zucchini noodles and steam noodles until soft
2. In a food processor mix the remaining ingredients and process until smooth
3. When ready, serve noodles with sauce

Serves: **4**

Prep Time: **10** Minutes

Cook Time: **30** Minutes

Total Time: **40** Minutes

INGREDIENTS

- 1 butternut squash
- 1 tablespoon olive oil
- ½ cup bacon
- ½ cup cashews
- 1 clove garlic
- ½ cup almond milk
- ½ tsp salt
- ¼ tsp pepper
- ½ cup peas
- 1 tablespoon parsley

DIRECTIONS

1. Preheat the oven to 375 F
2. Spiralize butternut squash into noodles
3. Place on a baking sheet and toss with olive oil

4. Bake for 8-10 minutes

5. In a bowl mix remaining, except peas, and place in a blender, blend until smooth

6. Pour the sauce into a skillet with peas, add butternut squash pasta and toss to coat

7. Top with parsley and serve

Serves: **5**

Prep Time: **10** Minutes

Cook Time: **30** Minutes

Total Time: **40** Minutes

INGREDIENTS

- 1 box gluten-free linguini
- 1 tablespoon garlic-infused olive oil
- 3 tablespoons butter
- 1 lb. shrimp
- 1 tsp Italian seasoning
- ½ tsp red pepper flakes
- 3 cups spinach
- juice of ½ lemon
- 1 tablespoon parsley

DIRECTIONS

1. Cook pasta according to package instructions
2. Drain and toss with olive oil
3. In a pot add shrimp and cook in melted butter

4. Add red pepper flakes, Italian seasoning, spinach and cook until done

5. Add shrimp to pasta mixture, top with lemon juice, herbs, pepper and serve

THANK YOU FOR READING THIS BOOK!

Printed in Great Britain
by Amazon